Internal Force Fitness: Everyday Exercise Routine 1

By Richard Neville

Distributed by:

Internal Force Fitness
www.internalforcefitness.co.uk

About the Internal Force Fitness: Everyday Exercise Routine 1

Internal Force Fitness are pleased to offer for the first time an English language version of the famous Chinese 'gymnastics' routine practised by Primary and High School students across China.

With its roots in Tai Chi and Chi Kung, this routine is an ideal everyday workout.

Complete list of movements:

1. Stand
2. The March
3. 12:15
4. 12:45
5. Double Draw
6. Windmill
7. The Wizard
8. Double Draw (Right)
9. Windmill (Right)
10. The Wizard (Right)
Repeat 3 - 10
11. Chicken Wing
12. Chicken Wing (Right)
13. Monk
14. Fly-By
Repeat 11 - 14
15. Swim (2 reps)
16. Pull & Pogo (2 reps)
17. Draw the Bow (left)
18. Swim (2 reps)
19. Pull & Pogo (2 reps)
20. Draw the Bow (right)
Repeat 15 - 20
21. The Cape
22. The Cape (right side)
23. Bowling
24. Bowling (right side)
Repeat 21 - 24
25. Cross-Kick (kick with right leg)
26. Cross-Kick (kick with left leg)
27. Balance (touch left foot twice)
28. Balance (touch right foot twice)
Repeat 25 - 28

29. Step-Reach-Toe-Squat (anti-clockwise)
30. Step-Reach-Toe-Squat (clockwise)
31. Up tempo (optional)
32. Floating
33. Tap front and back
34. Gather in the energy

Stand

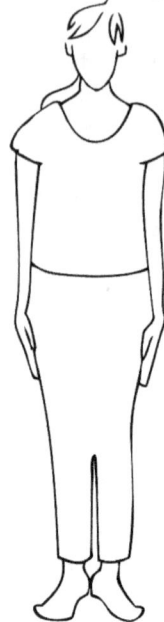

Fig. 1. Stand

STAND

Stand with your feet hip-width apart and your knees slightly bent (Fig.1). Arms are down by your sides with fingers pointing down and palms flat against the thighs.

Stand up straight by tilting the pelvis forwards slightly, and lifting your chest by pulling your shoulders back.

Tip: To tilt your pelvis, put your hands on either side of your hips – fingers on your butt cheeks, thumbs on the front of the hips. Turn your hands clockwise and turn the pelvis at the same time (it won't turn very far). You will feel your entire posture change. Now unclench your buttocks, but stay in the position! (If you did this without sub-consciously clenching your buttocks – well done)

This is also an excellent stand alone exercise: simply repeat a dozen or so times, alternating between relaxing and standing tall. For the purposes of this routine however, you should keep standing tall for the entire routine.

The March

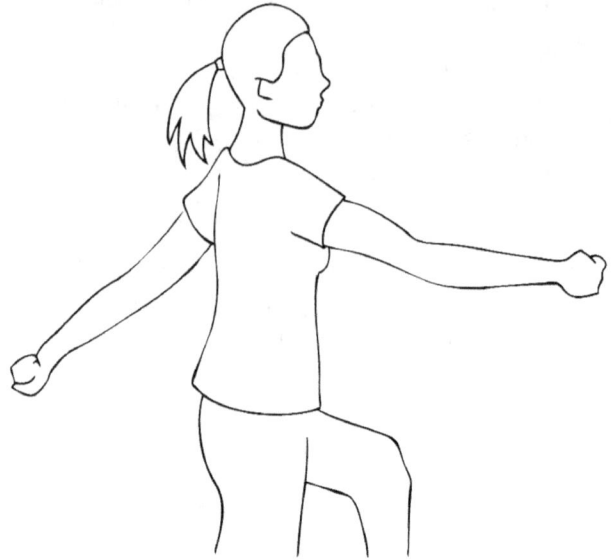

Fig. 2. The March

THE MARCH

Stand with your feet hip-width apart and your knees slightly bent (Fig.1). Arms are down by your sides with the fists lightly clenched. Starting with the **left** leg, lift your knee, then your ankle, then your heel, then your toes. Lifting the toes 2-3 inches from the floor is sufficient – do not raise the knee more than waist height.

At the same time swing the **right** arm forwards, and the left arm backwards. Keep the upper body straight and keep control of the arms. (In other words don't twist your body to get your arms to go higher, and don't let them swing above neck height.) 45 degrees from the body front and back is sufficient – but the overall aim is simply to have the arms swing an equal distance from the body in both directions.

Now reverse the process by bringing the toe, ankle, and knee back to the ground and the arms back to the sides, fists still lightly clenched. Without pausing, repeat the moves by lifting the **right** leg and swinging the **left** arm forward so you are marching on the spot.

Raise both legs 8 times each.

Tip: Count every time you swing your **right** arm forwards – when you reach 8, you're done!

Stand with your feet hip-width apart and your knees slightly bent (Fig. 1). Arms are down by your sides with fingers pointing down and palms flat against the thighs. (After finishing the March, simply take a breath, open your hands and continue straight into this move.)

Step out to your **left** so your feet are slightly wider than shoulder-width apart. At the same time raise your arms out to the sides to shoulder level. Fingertips are pointing away from you and palms are facing down.

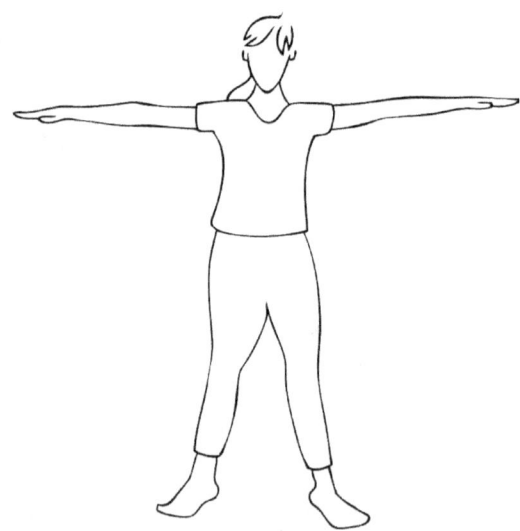

Fig. 3. Step out into cross

Hands only: Leaving your first and second fingers pointing forward, curl the third and little finger into the palm and place the thumb on top of them. Both hands adopt this pose during this and the next 4 exercises.

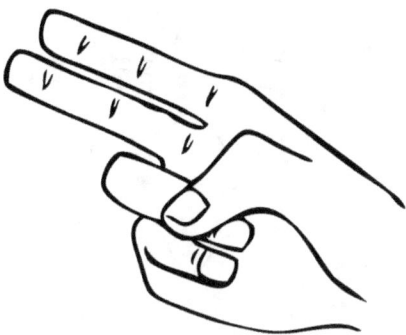

Fig. 3a. Hand position

With hands as above, raise the **left** arm up to the sky. Palm facing forward. At the same time raise the right arm straight to the sky, but then continue the arc by bending the elbow until the fingertips of the right hand have ran down the left forearm and are level with (and in front of) the elbow of the left arm. Palm facing forward.

Tip the head back as your lifting your arms until you are looking at the sky where the fingertips of the left hand are pointing.

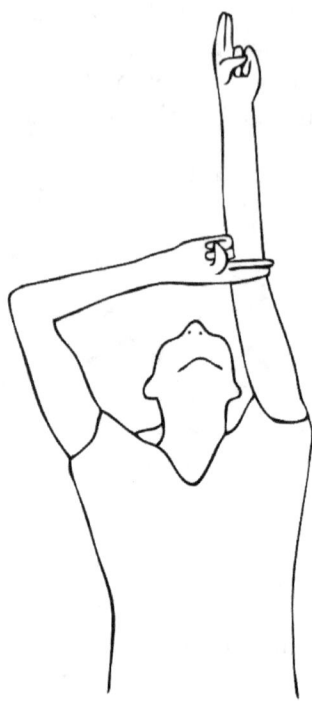

Fig. 3b. 12:15

Straighten the right arm, tip head back down, and lower both arms together to the starting point (star shape). Open your hands as you lower your arms to your sides and step in left foot to right foot. You are now back where you started.

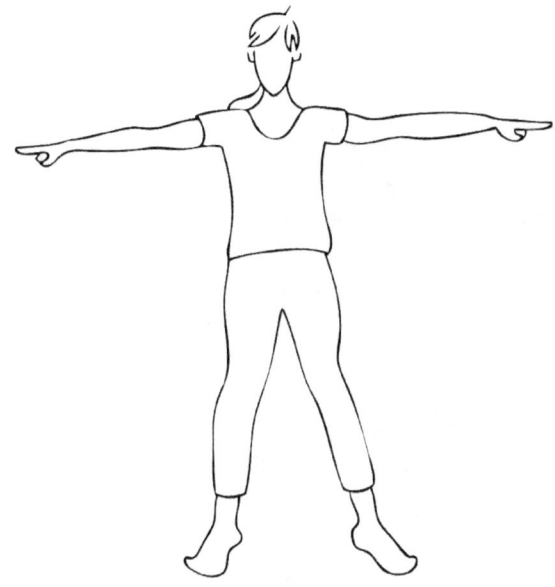

Fig. 3c. Cross with bent fingers

Note: 12:15 relates to the position of your arms when you are in the final position.

Tip: The easiest way to differentiate between this move and the 12:45 is to remember that if you are stepping out on your **left** foot; your **left** arm is straight and vice versa.

12:45

The opposite of the 12:15. Step out onto the **right** foot, and straighten the **right** arm. The left arm bends at the elbow. Finish by stepping in right foot to left foot and lowering your arms to your sides.

The 12:15 and the 12:45 are performed as follows:

Step out and raise arms to shoulder height.
Curl fingers.
Raise arms and look up.
Lower arms to shoulder height.
Open fingers and step in.

Double Draw

Stand with your feet hip-width apart and your knees slightly bent (Fig.1). Arms are down by your sides with fingers pointing down and palms flat against the thighs. (After finishing the 12:45, simply take a breath, and continue straight into this move.)

Take a half-step forward on your **left** foot 45 degrees to your left. Your left foot will be on a diagonal – not straight.

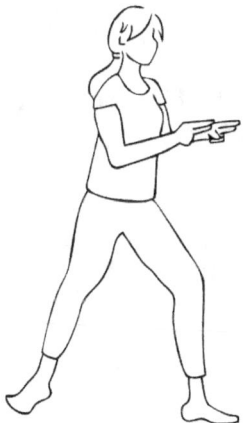

Fig. 4. Double Draw

Lift both hands vertically up the body until they are at waist height and at the same time curl the fingers as in Fig. 3a. Turn the hands 45 degrees so they are now facing forwards, palms are facing inwards. Dynamically thrust both hands forward until the arms are straight.

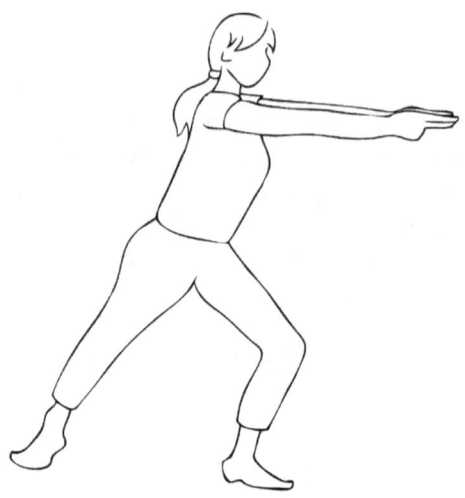

Fig. 4a. Double Draw (Completed)

Lean forward slightly so your left knee is over your left toes and you feel a slight stretch in your right leg. (If you don't feel a stretch, don't worry – it just means you are already nice and loose.)

Windmill

Staying in this position, keep the left arm straight and make a big clockwise circle with the **right** arm bringing the arm as close to the right ear as possible. Palm is facing away from you the whole time (Turn hand around anti-clockwise as you start and back as you finish).

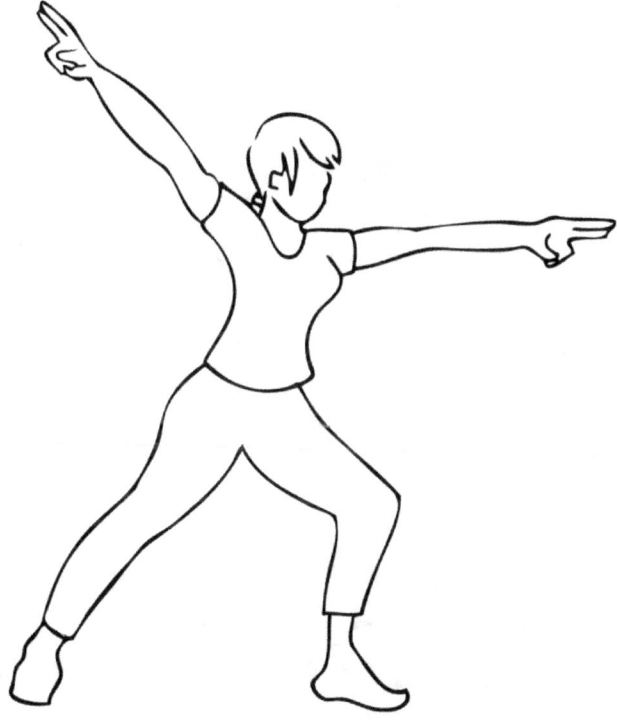

Fig. 5. Windmill

The Wizard

Still keeping the left arm straight, begin to make another clockwise circle with the **right** arm. When the right hand gets to about the height of the top of your head, pull the arm backwards (the forearm will be horizontal) until the right hand is just above the head. The right palm will be facing away from you. Keep the right elbow as high as possible.

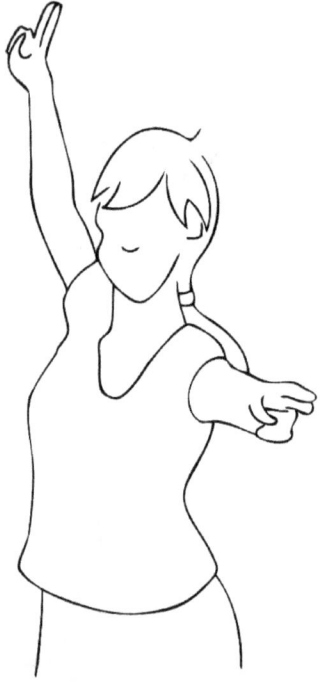

Fig. 6. The Wizard (Front view)

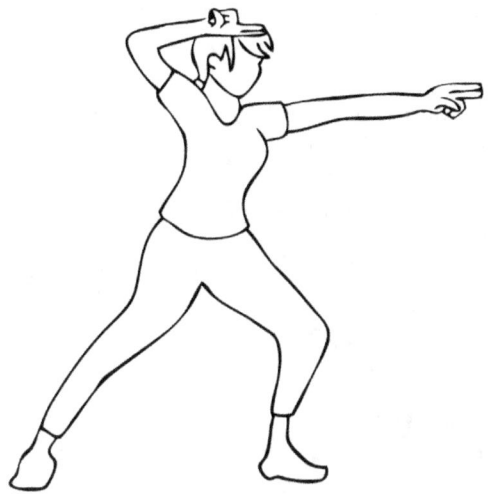

Fig. 6a. The Wizard (Side view)

Open both hands and lower the arms to the sides as you step in left foot to right foot.

Double Draw – Right

Take a half-step forward on your **right** foot 45 degrees to your right. The rest of this movement is exactly the same as the left side.

Windmill - Right

Keep the right arm straight and make the circle with the left arm.

The Wizard – Right

Keep the right arm straight and pull the left arm back.

Open both hands and lower the arms to the sides as you step in right foot to left foot.

Tip: When you step out on your **left**, it is the **right** arm that moves, and vice versa.

Repeat the following 1 more time in order:

12:15
12:45
Double Draw (Left)
Windmill (Left)
The Wizard (Left)
Double Draw (Right)
Windmill (Right)
The Wizard (Right)

Chicken Wing

Stand with your feet hip-width apart and your knees slightly bent (Fig.1). Arms are down by your sides with fingers pointing down and palms flat against the thighs. (After finishing The Wizard, simply take a breath, and continue straight into this move.)

Step out to your **left** so your feet are slightly wider than shoulder-width apart. At the same time raise your **left** elbow to shoulder height. Your left forearm is horizontal and your left hand in just in front of your **right** shoulder. Palm is facing down. Look to your **left** as you are stepping out and raising your arm.

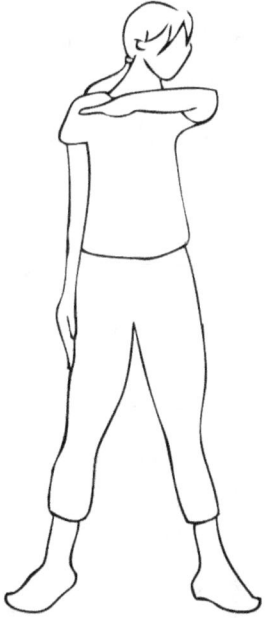

Fig. 7. Chicken Wing

The right arm does not move.

Keeping the arms in this position, turn the head to look forwards, then back to the left, then back to the front as you lower the arms and step in left to right.

The Chicken Wing is performed as follows:

Step out and raise the arm while looking in the direction of the arm being raised.
Look forward.
Look back to the raised arm.
Look forward as you lower the arm and step in.

Chicken Wing – Right

As above, but this time step out onto the **right**, and raise the **right** elbow.

Monk

Stand with your feet hip-width apart and your knees slightly bent (Fig.1). Arms are down by your sides with fingers pointing down and palms flat against the thighs. (After finishing The Chicken Wing on the right side, simply take a breath, and continue straight into this move.)

With both hands behind the back, place the back of the open right hand against the palm of the open left hand (making a cross shape). Lightly press both hands against the small of the back.

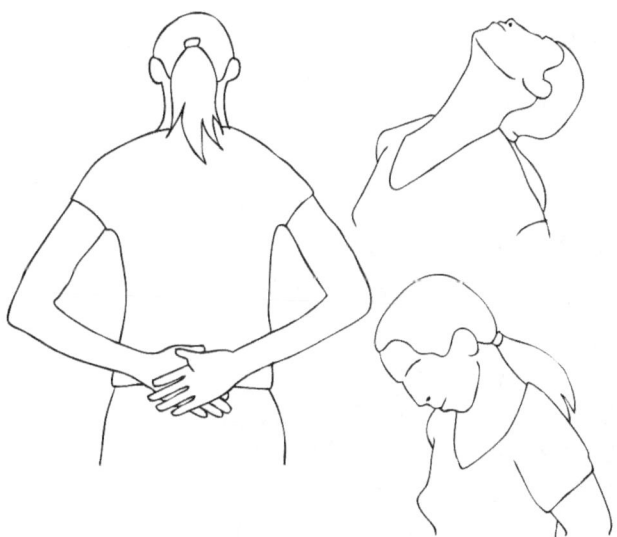

Fig. 8. Monk & Fly-By

Without bending your spine lower your head to your chest by bending your neck.

Lift the head back up until it is back in the starting position.

Tip: The aim is simply to touch your chest with your chin.

Without pausing go straight into;

Fly-By

From the upright position keep raising the chin until you are looking up at the sky/ceiling.

Return to the starting position.

Tip: Your eyes should follow an imaginary aeroplane as it appears on the horizon in front of you until it flies overhead.

Note: Only go as far as your **neck** will let you – there is nothing to be gained by leaning forwards or backwards to get extra distance.
Repeat the following 1 more time in order:

Chicken Wing
Chicken Wing – Right
Monk (Left hand against palm of right hand this time)
Fly-By

Swim

Stand with your feet hip-width apart and your knees slightly bent (Fig.1). Arms are down by your sides with fingers pointing down and palms flat against the thighs. (After finishing Fly-By, simply take a breath and continue straight into this move.)

Bring the hands together in the centre of the body, 5-10cm from the chest. Fingers are extended and pointing forwards.

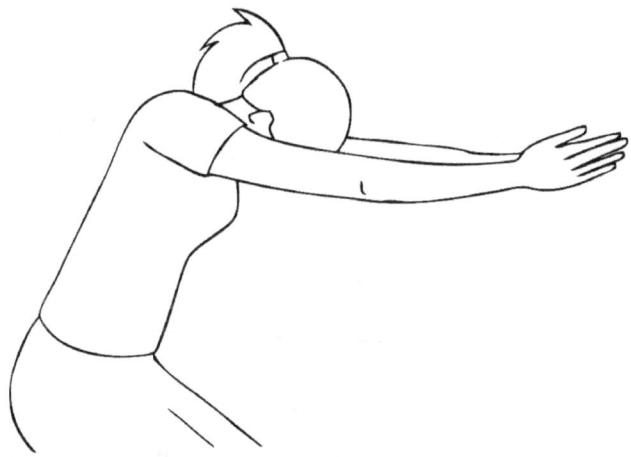

Fig. 9. Swim

Bending the knees slightly extend the arms dynamically forward as far as possible (as if you were swimming). Look down through the arms to the floor. Your upper body should bend forward as far as is comfortable while keeping your balance.

At the furthest point, pull the hands apart and turn them each 90 degrees so the palms are facing away from the body. As you raise the upper body and straighten the knees pull both arms backwards as though you are trying to propel yourself through water.

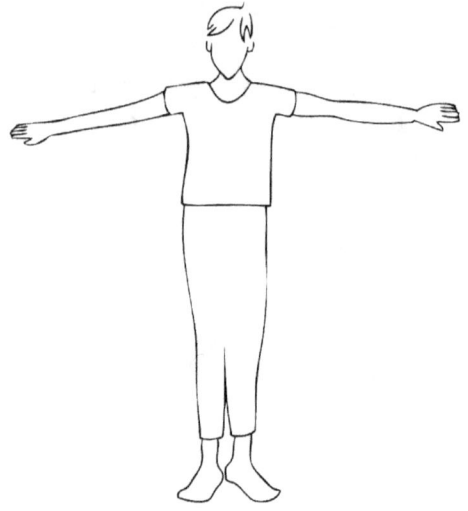

Fig. 9a. Propel

When your arms reach their natural resistance point (don't force them behind you more than they will naturally go), your fingers should now be pointing backwards and your palms facing each other.

Turn the fingers down and around so they are facing forwards again (move the arms to whatever extent is necessary to do this). Following the line of an imaginary 'V' shape, bring the hands together in the starting position and repeat immediately 1 more time.

Finish with hands together in front of the body.

Pull & Pogo

At the end of the 2nd repetition of Swim, keep the fingertips of the middle fingers touching and open the hands like a hinge so the palms are now facing down. Hands are chest height 5-10cm in front of the chest and forearms are horizontal.

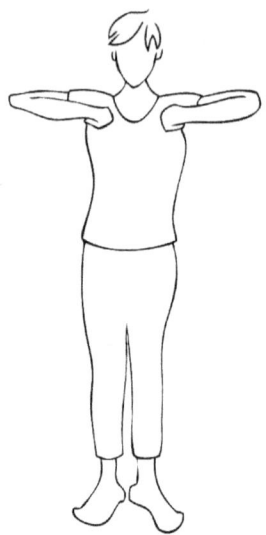

Fig. 10. Pull & Pogo

Make fists (palms are still facing down). Pull your elbows back as far as possible (pull) while at the same time bending your knees 45 degrees (pogo). Stand up straight and return fists to start position. Keep fists clenched and repeat immediately 1 more time.

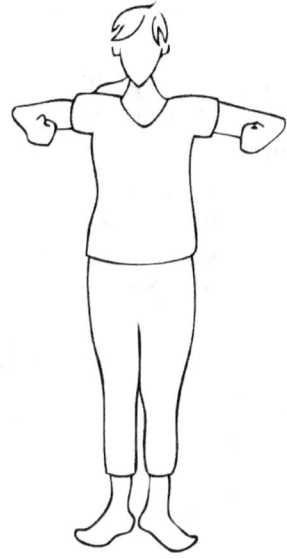

Fig. 10a. Pull & Pogo

Tip: While this is a dynamic movement, focus on trying to make your shoulder blades meet, not just flinging your elbows back.

Draw the Bow

From the final 'make fist' position at the end of the second repetition of Pull and Pogo, step out on the **left** foot to slightly wider than shoulder width apart. At the same time extend the **right** arm out to your right side on a diagonal skywards, and extend the left hand in the same direction. Turn the fists so the thumbs are pointing upwards. The left arm follows the diagonal of the right arm. The left fist should come to around right wrist level, but don't worry if you can't stretch that far. Look up to the right hand.

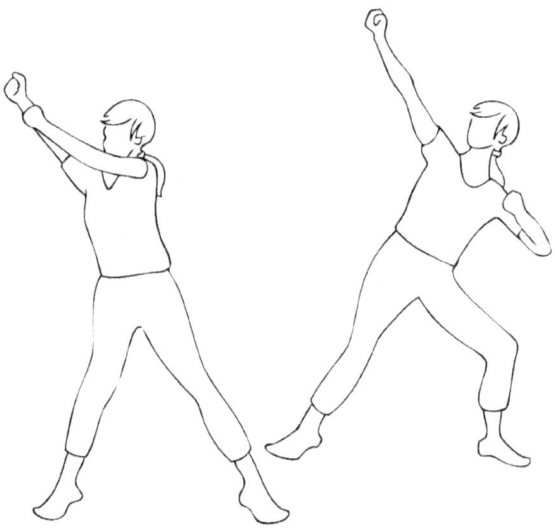

Fig. 11. Draw the Bow

Tip: Imagine you have a bow in your right hand and you are preparing to fire an arrow into the sky.

Keeping the right arm where it is, and the right leg straight, pull back on the 'bow' string with the left hand and bend the left knee slightly. Your left hand should end up just below your left shoulder.

Straighten the left leg as you lower both arms to the sides.

Repeat the following 1 more time in order:

- Swim (Two repetitions)
- Pull & Pogo (Two repetitions)
- Draw the Bow (Right side – step out on the right foot and raise the left arm in a high diagonal and pull back with the right hand)

Now repeat the entire sequence 1 more time:

- Swim (2 reps)
- Pull & Pogo (2 reps)
- Draw the Bow (left)
- Swim (2 reps)
- Pull & Pogo (2 reps)
- Draw the Bow (right)

The Cape

Stand with your feet hip-width apart and your knees slightly bent (Fig.1). Arms are down by your sides with fingers pointing down and palms flat against the thighs.

Step out to your **left** so your feet are slightly wider than shoulder-width apart. At the same time raise your arms out to the sides to shoulder level (Fig. 3.). Fingertips are pointing away from you and palms are facing down. Keep the pelvis 'tucked in' (tilted forward), and bend the knees a little further than normal. Make fists with both hands.

As if you are 'swishing' a cape, turn your entire upper body to the left as far as possible.

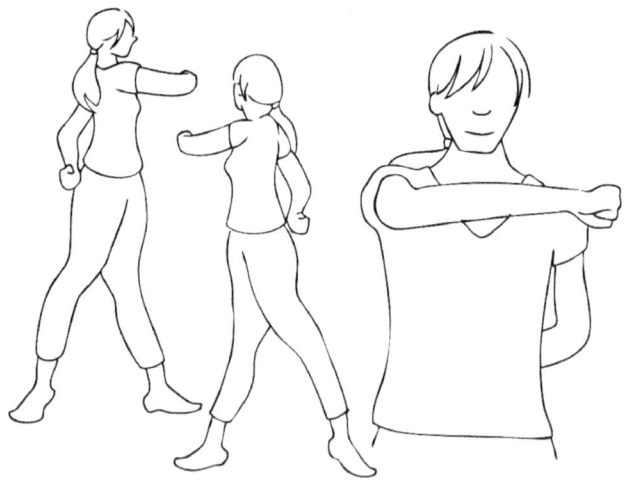

Fig. 12. The Cape

Tip: Keeping your knees bent a little more than usual will ensure you only turn the upper body. It will also protect your knees from being twisted. Don't be surprised or disappointed if this stops you from being able to turn very far. That is entirely normal.

The right arm: The right arm stays straight until you reach the furthest point then bend the arm at the elbow so the first knuckle of the right fist is approx 10cm from the front of the left shoulder. Right elbow is kept high.

The left arm: At the same time the left arm stays straight until you reach the furthest point, but as you turn it drops on a 45 degree angle. At the furthest point the arm bends at the elbow until the back of the left fist comes to rest on the small of the back.

Tip: Aim for a nice smooth rhythmic action by keeping the shoulders loose.

Return to the starting (cross) position, and then step in left foot to right foot, lowering the arms.

The Cape (right side).

Step out onto your right foot, and turn your upper body to the right. Your left hand comes to your right shoulder and your right hand rests on your lower back.

Return to the starting (cross) position, and then step in right foot to left foot.

Bowling

Stand with your feet hip-width apart and your knees slightly bent (Fig.1). Arms are down by your sides with fingers pointing down and palms flat against the thighs.

Step out to your **left** so your feet are slightly wider than shoulder-width apart. At the same time raise your arms out to the sides to shoulder level (Fig. 3.). Fingertips are pointing away from you and palms are facing down.

Keeping all of your weight on your **left** leg, bring your right leg as far backwards and to the left as possible without twisting the pelvis.

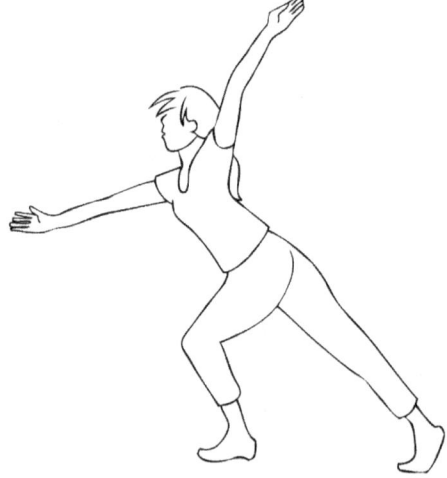

Fig. 13. Bowling (Side view)

At the same time push the right hand forward, palm up, fingers pointing forwards, as though you have just bowled a bowling ball.

As the right arm goes forward the left arm should naturally come backwards, and will rise slightly to around head height. Palm stays down and fingers point backwards.

Reverse the process and return to the cross position. Lower the arms and step in left foot to right foot.

Tip: Whichever leg you step back with, that is the arm that goes forwards.

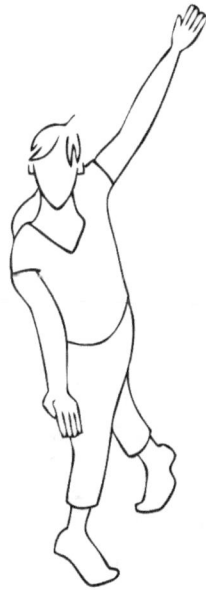

Fig. 13a. Bowling (Front view)

Bowling (right side).

Without pausing, step out onto your right. Step backwards with your left leg and 'bowl' with your right hand.

Repeat the following 1 more time in order:

The Cape
The Cape (right side)
Bowling
Bowling (right side)

Cross-Kick

Stand with your feet hip-width apart and your knees slightly bent (Fig.1). Arms are down by your sides with fingers pointing down and palms flat against the thighs.

Take a comfortable step forward on your **left** foot. At the same time make an 'X' with your forearms about 30cm in front of your chest. Your left forearm is closest to you.

As you are raising your arms, make fists – palms facing the body.

Dynamically swing the arms backwards opening the hands and extending the fingers as you do so. Palms will be facing away from one another and fingers pointing back.

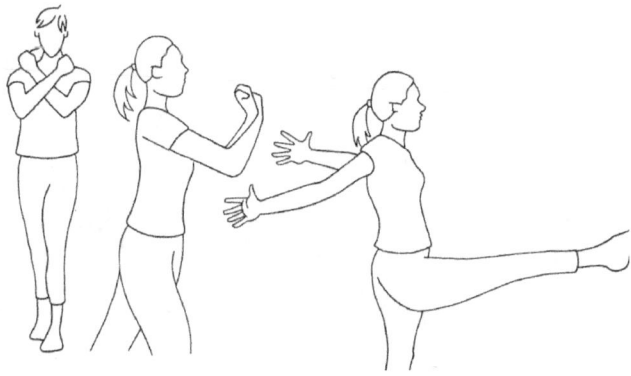

Fig. 14. Cross Kick

As you are swinging your arms backwards kick to the front with a straight **right** leg and pointed toes. Kick as high as you can while keeping your balance – knee height is fine.

Reverse the entire process to get back into the starting position:

Lower the leg
Re-Cross the arms
Step back on the left leg
Lower the arms

Cross-Kick (right side)

Without pausing, step out onto your right. Step forward on your right foot and kick with your left.

Tip: Kick as if you were kicking a ball.

Balance

Stand with your feet hip-width apart and your knees slightly bent (Fig.1). Arms are down by your sides with fingers pointing down and palms flat against the thighs.

Raise the **left** arm only to shoulder height, fingers pointing away from you and palm pointing down.

Lift the left leg until it is high enough for you to touch the foot with your **right** hand. Lift the leg on a vertical line. To touch the foot, move the right hand across the centre of the body.

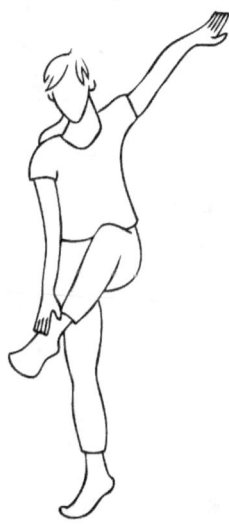

Fig. 15. Balance

Lower the left leg and raise the right arm to shoulder height (matching the left – you are now in Fig. 3. position).

Lift the left leg again and lower the right arm in an arc to touch it again. Lower the leg and raise the arm again.

Now raise the right leg and lower the left arm in an arc to touch the right foot. Return and repeat on this side 1 more time.

Lower arms back to the sides.

Repeat the following 1 more time in order:

Cross-Kick (kick with right leg)
Cross-Kick (kick with left leg)
Balance (touch left foot twice)
Balance (touch right foot twice)

Step-Reach-Toe-Squat

Stand with your feet hip-width apart and your knees slightly bent (Fig.1). Arms are down by your sides with fingers pointing down and palms flat against the thighs. (After finishing Balance, simply take a breath and continue straight into this move.)

Take a half-step forward on your **left** foot 45 degrees to your left. Your left foot will be on a diagonal – not straight.

At the same time swing both arms up into the air so they are pointing straight up. Lean backwards a little if you are able. Your entire upper body is pointing the same direction as your left foot.

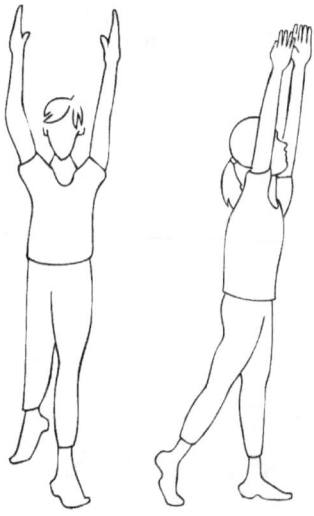

Fig. 16. Step and Reach

Tip: Adjust your back (right) foot as much as is necessary to stop you twisting your knee.

Tip: As you become more comfortable with this move, you might want to step out onto your left toes, stretch up and back a little and then flatten your foot. You will feel the stretch in your abs.

Step forwards with your **right** foot so you are now standing 45 degrees to the left of your original starting position and with your feet just over shoulder width apart.

As you are stepping, bend forwards at the waist and lower the arms to touch your toes. Keep your legs straight if you can. Keeping the legs straight and not being able to touch the toes is more important than bending the knees to touch them.

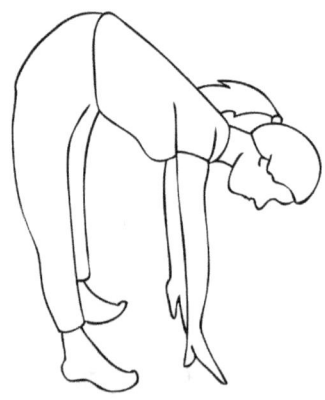

Fig. 17. Toe

Come part of the way back up and rest the hands just above the knees – fingers pointing towards each other. Bring the **right** foot in to meet the left, then bend the knees fully and go into a squat position. You may raise your heels if you wish.

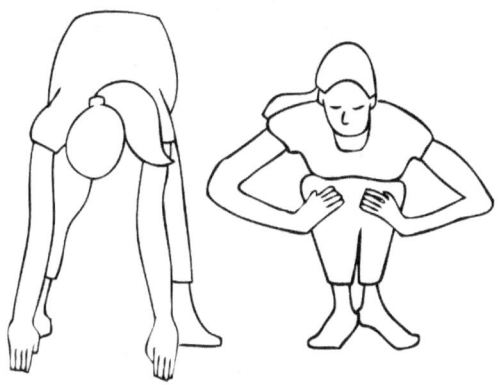

Fig. 18. Squat

Stand.

From where you are now, step out on the left foot again at a 45 degree angle and repeat the entire sequence.

Repeat 2 more times which should bring you back more or less to the starting position.

Tip: Think of stepping out to corners of a square

Step-Reach-Toe-Squat (clockwise)

Repeat the sequence 4 more times only this time going in the other direction. Step out on the right foot, follow through with the left. Step in left to right when you crouch/squat.

Tip: Do not feel like the transitions needs to be seamless between these moves. You can move around as much as you like.

Up-Tempo section (Optional)

Stand with your feet hip-width apart and your knees slightly bent (Fig.1). Arms are down by your sides with fingers pointing down and palms flat against the thighs. (After finishing Step-Reach-Toe-Squat, simply take a breath and continue straight into this move.)

Jog 3 paces forward, lifting the left arm and right leg first. Fists are slightly clenched. Try and touch your butt with your heels.

Land with your feet hip width apart and arms down by your sides.

Jump a little in to the air and open your legs slightly, so that when you land they are shoulder width apart.

At the same time bring hands up the centre of the body, lift elbows and make fists. Hands pause at chest height 5-10cm in front of the chest and 5-10cm apart. Forearms are horizontal.

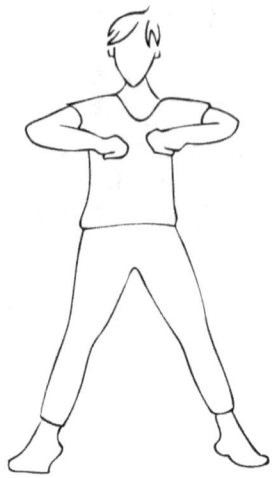

Fig. 19. Up tempo - Elbows

Jump again and reverse the move, bringing the feet together and lowering the arms.

Jump a little in to the air and open your legs slightly, so that when you land they are shoulder width apart.

At the same time raise the arms and clap the hands above the head. (This is the same as a traditional 'Jumping Jack')

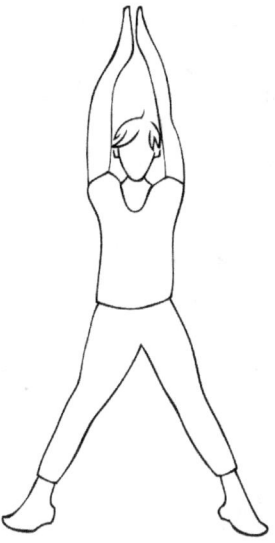

Fig. 19b. Up tempo – Jumping Jack

Jump again and reverse the move, bringing the feet together and lowering the arms.

Jog 3 paces backwards and repeat the entire sequence 1 more time.

Tip: If your workout space does not allow for jumping around, simply march 3 steps forward (or on the spot), and step out to the left (then the right) and complete the moves that way. It is also acceptable to miss this sequence out of your daily routine.

Floating

Stand with your feet hip-width apart and your knees slightly bent (Fig.1). Arms are down by your sides with fingers pointing down and palms flat against the thighs.

Step out to your **left** so your feet are slightly wider than shoulder-width apart. At the same time raise your arms out to the sides to shoulder level (Fig.3). Fingertips are pointing away from you and palms are facing down.

Putting all the weight onto your left leg, slowly and gently lower the arms back your sides while at the same time 'floating' the right leg over to meet the left. Raise the arms again as you step back out on the right, then putting all of the weight on your right foot, drop the arms and float the left leg over to the right.

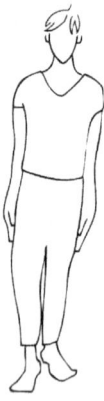

Fig. 20. Floating

Float the right leg to the left one more time, then step back onto the right with arms raised. Step in left foot to right foot (normally) and lower the arms.

Full sequence:

Step out onto left
Float right to left
Return
Left to right
Return
Right to left
Return
Step in left to right

Tap front and back

Stand with your feet hip-width apart and your knees slightly bent (Fig.1). Arms are down by your sides with fingers pointing down and palms flat against the thighs.

Step out to your **left** so your feet are slightly wider than shoulder-width apart. At the same time raise your arms out to the sides to shoulder level (Fig.3). Fingertips are pointing away from you and palms are facing down. Keep the pelvis 'tucked in' (tilted forward), and bend the knees a little further than normal.

Turn your shoulders as far to the left as you can without twisting the pelvis, keeping the arms outstretched.

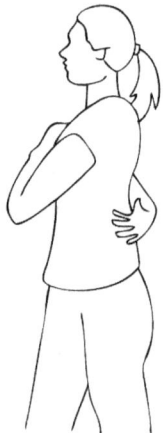

Fig. 21. Tap Front and Back

At the furthest point, bend the right arm and tap your left shoulder. At the same time drop your left arm enough to tap the base of your spine with the back of your left hand.

Tip: Aim for a nice smooth rhythmic action by keeping the shoulders loose.

Return to the starting (cross) position, and then step in left foot to right foot, lowering the arms.

Repeat by stepping out onto the right foot and touching the right shoulder with the left hand and the spine with the right hand.

Return to the starting (cross) position, and then step in right foot to left foot, lowering the arms.

Step out onto the left one more time, raising the arms as before. Turn to the left, but this time keep both arms loose and touch the left **hip** with the right hand and the right hip with the back of the left hand.

Return to the starting (cross) position, and then step in left foot to right foot, lowering the arms.

Tip: Keeping your knees bent a little more than usual will ensure you only turn the upper body. It will also protect your knees from being twisted. Don't be surprised or disappointed if this stops you from being able to turn very far. That is entirely normal.

Full sequence:

Step out onto left

Turn left and touch and tap
Step in
Step out onto right
Turn right and touch and tap
Step in
Step out onto left
Turn left and touch and tap – low
Step in left to right

Repeat the following 1 more time in order:

Floating (Step out onto right side first)

Full sequence:

Step out onto right
Float left to right
Return
Right to left
Return
Left to right
Return
Step in right to left

Tap front and back (turn to the right first)

Full sequence:

Step out onto right
Turn right and touch and tap
Step in
Step out onto left
Turn left and touch and tap

Step in
Step out onto right
Turn right and touch and tap – low
Step in right to left

Gather in the Energy (Chi)

Stand with your feet hip-width apart and your knees slightly bent (Fig.1). Arms are down by your sides with fingers pointing down and palms flat against the thighs.

Step out onto the left foot so your feet are shoulder width apart.

Turn the hands away from the body so the palms are facing up. Raise both arms in an arc up the side of the body until they are pointing to the sky, collecting the 'energy' around you as you lift them. Look up to the hands, fingers pointing to the sky. Bring the thumbs and fingers together and then turn the hands and point them downwards (create a 'diamond shape' between your hands). Bring the collected energy down by lowering the hands down the centre of the body, pausing at the belly button. Follow your hands with your eyes. Open the hands (release the energy into your system) and repeat 1 more time.

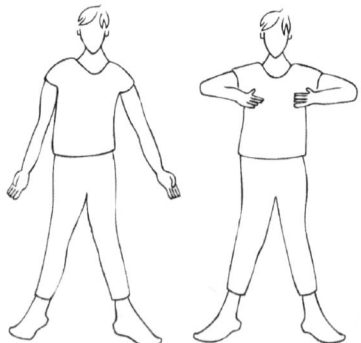

Fig. 22. Gather in the Energy

Step in left foot to right foot.

Conclusion

The **Internal Force Fitness: Everyday Exercise Routine** is designed to wake your body up and give all of the major muscle groups a good stretch. It is a routine for every day of your life, wherever you may be.

Once you have mastered the full routine you might like to join your local Tai Chi club, as this routine owes a lot to the slow and deliberate Tai Chi forms.

www.internalforcefitness.co.uk

www.ingramcontent.com/pod-product-compliance
Lightning Source LLC
Chambersburg PA
CBHW060228290526
45789CB00003B/1456